FOLLOWING DIRECTIONS

SIX-MINUTE THINKING SKILLS

WORKBOOK 1

INTRODUCTION

Welcome to the ***Six-Minute Thinking Skills*** series. These workbooks are designed for busy parents and teachers who need easy-to-use and effective materials for working with learners who struggle with the thinking skills required for school success.

This workbook, ***Following Directions,*** provides step-by-step activities to quickly build the ability to independently follow multi-step directions.

Key details of this workbook are:

- Suitable for 1-1 or classroom use

  This book can be used in a classroom or with a single learner. No group work is required, though the Coaching section provides suggestions for including pair and group work.

- Includes a wide variety of tasks

The workbook includes more than one hundred activities covering thirty-four different question types. Tasks vary from day to day so students are always engaged with new instructions.

The wide variety of tasks develops your student's flexibility in dealing with many different types of directions.

- Gradually increments difficulty

Each of the thirty-four question types includes multiple examples which gradually increase in difficulty. Learners begin with simple steps, but will soon be interpreting information, creating rules, comparing data and defending decisions.

- Multi-purpose: Can be used to improve listening comprehension

Many children have trouble following multi-step oral instructions. If your learner has listening comprehension challenges, use the exercises in this book to quickly improve their skill. See the Coaching section for further information.

- No-prep. No extra materials required

Everything needed is included in the book - except for a pencil or pen! The student can write their answers in the book, or use a piece of paper if the book needs to be reused later.

- Small chunks. Use any time

Our worksheets are designed for 'six-minute sessions.' Anytime you have a spare moment, your learner can complete a worksheet and make progress.

INTRODUCTION

The ability to follow multi-step directions is key for school and learning success. Support your struggling learners with this fun, engaging workbook that will build your learner's ability and confidence in this important skill.

HOW TO COACH A SIX-MINUTE SESSION

Follow these suggestions for quick progress that will motivate your learners.

1. Have a consistent and regular schedule.

Consistency and regularity are important if you want to reach a goal. So, choose a regular schedule for your six-minute sessions, get your learner's agreement and stick to it! In a school setting, make this task a regular part of your students' day. In a home setting, aim for 3-4 times per week.

2. Devise a reward system.

Working on skill deficits is hard work for any learner. Appreciate your student's effort by building in a reward system. This may include a reward when a specific number of exercises are finished, when directions are completed correctly on the first try, or whatever will encourage your learner at this point in their journey. Remember to reward based on effort as well as correctness.

3. Don't answer questions except to explain the meaning of a word.

We want our learners to develop independence in following directions. So, right from the beginning expect this independence. Apart from explaining unfamiliar words, ask them to do their best and complete the task.

4. Include time for review and correction.

After your student has completed the activity, review your student's work. When identifying an error, make a positive statement and then provide the least information needed for the learner to make a correction. For example, prefer

> *Nice job. I can see most of your answer is correct, but there is also a small problem. Can you find it and fix it?*

to

> *You forgot to do the last instruction.*

The first method develops the student's ability to review their work and find the error. This valuable skill will lead to fewer errors in future worksheets.

Make sure that your learner always has a chance to physically correct their work.

5. Don't be afraid to repeat.

In the six-minute series, we have broken skill development into tiny steps. But even so, your learner may not master these skills instantly. Don't be afraid to create additional variants of a particular challenge until your learner develops confidence. The difficulty of the activities does increase through the book, so make sure your learner is successful before moving on.

If you are concerned about boredom, mix your review in with new lessons. In any case, don't move too far ahead if your learner still needs help with earlier skills.

6. Include listening skills.

Many of the activities in this book can be delivered orally instead of in writing. This is an excellent way to improve listening skills quickly.

Before delivering an oral instruction, make sure your learners have paper and a writing instrument ready to go. For shorter instructions, we suggest you give the whole instruction and repeat it once. For longer instructions, you may want to give one instruction at a time with a single repeat of each.

For added challenge with an exercise that is within your learner's skillset, change up the exercise details and only say the instruction once.

6. Make use of multiple learners.

If you are using this book in a small group or classroom setting, get the learners to review each other's worksheets. This will build excellent reviewing skills. Teach your learners to provide minimal information when identifying an error so that each student gets practice at finding errors in their own work.

For added benefit, you can also assign students to work in pairs or small groups to complete the activities.

8. CALENDAR

Draw a hat on the day that comes two days after July 16. Draw a sun on the day before July 30. How many days between the two pictures?

JULY

		1	2	3	4	5
6	7	8	9	10	11	12
13	14	15	16	17	18	19
20	21	22	23	24	25	26
27	28	29	30	31		

9. FORMS

Read the paragraph and fill in the form below.

My name is Fiona Dumont and I live in California. I was born on February 16th, 2008. My favorite sport is baseball. My mom's name is Cathy Belton and my Dad's name is Greg Dumont. I am visiting the doctor today to get my eyes checked. My mom thinks I might need glasses. Afterwards, we are going swimming at our local pool.

Name: _____

Date of Birth: _____

Mother's Name: _____

Father's Name: _____

Reason for Visit: _____

10. ADD TO

Copy the following sentence below, but change the location. Next add another three sentences to continue the story.

Hallie wandered into the creepy mansion.

11 DESCRIPTION

Think about your favorite food. Write a description about it that is at least 3 sentences. Keep going if you have more to say.

12. DIRECTIONS

Use the space below. Write your name in the top left hand corner. In the middle, draw a circle. Write the number 6 below the circle and the number three above it.

13. IMAGINE

Your dad lost the car keys. Write a short story about how he lost the keys and found them again.

14. DRAW & DESCRIBE

Find something large in the room where you are. Draw a picture of it. Write 2 sentences about that object.

15. DRAW MAP

Draw a map of the room you are in. Include the furniture, doors and windows.

16. MOUSE

Write directions for how the mouse will get to the cheese. Use words like up, down, left, right and tell how many squares to move in each direction.

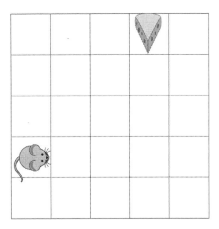

17. CATEGORIZE

Categorize these words into three columns. Put a heading at the top of each column to describe the words in each column.

Dog House Banana Orange Apartment Cat Rabbit Cabin Apple Bird Peach Mansion

18. LINES

Use the lines below. Write your favorite color on the third line. Write your birth month on the fifth line.

Write the numbers from 1 to 10 on the seventh line.

_____

_____

_____

_____

_____

_____

_____

19. COMPARISON

Look at the table below and write a sentence that describes what two fruits have in common (something the same.)

Now write a sentence that describes a difference between two fruits.

Fruit	Color
Apple	Red
Orange	Orange
Raspberry	Red
Banana	Yellow
Cherry	Red
Pineapple	Yellow

20. DISTRIBUTION

You have ten dollars to spend. Chips are $2 each and chocolate bars are $3 each.

What would you buy? List your purchases below with the price of each and the total cost.

Explain why you made these choices.

21. WORD PROBLEM

Read the word problem and then write the answer below. Write another word problem that includes buying something.

Jaxon bought two books for each of his two sisters. How many books did Jaxon buy?

22. RANDOM WORDS

Make a list of five random words. Now write five sentences below your list. Each sentence must contain two of your five words.

23. FIND THE PROBLEM

Which instruction is incorrect? Replace it with a correct instruction.

1. Draw a large box and shade it light grey.
2. Draw a smaller square inside the grey square.
3. Draw a lower case A inside the small square.

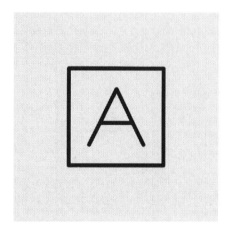

24. INFORMATION RETRIEVAL

Choose a country and write down four details about that country. Use bullet points for the details. Don't forget to title your list with the name of the country. At the end, note down if you have been to that country or not.

25. LETTERS

Write 5 letters down the left hand side of the space below. Each letter should be different - no repeats. Think of a food that starts with each letter and write the foods in a line at the bottom.

26. MAKE PATTERN

Write a number sequence that follows this rule.

Start at 2 and add 3.

Write each number on the line below. Stop when you have filled up the line.

--- --- --- --- --- --- ---

WACKY 1

Write the numbers one to ten upside down in the space below.

27. DRAW

Write step-by-step instructions for drawing these owl eyes.

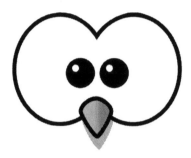

Test your instructions by reading them to someone who hasn't seen the drawing. If you need to, improve your directions.

28. CHANGES

Write out the number below, but make the following changes.
Replace all 8's with 1. Replace all 7's with 3.

5 8 3 8 9 1 7 5 3 2 7

- - - - - - - - - - -

Add the numbers that you wrote and write the total here.

29. SHAPES

Draw a horizontal line. Above the line, draw a circle that touches the
line. Draw a triangle inside the circle.

30. ALPHABET

List ten foods on the left hand side of the page. Now rewrite the list in alphabetical order on the right hand side of the page.

31. DRAWING

Draw a tree. Draw a chair under the tree. Write a sentence about the chair and the tree.

32. CREATE TABLE

Read the following paragraph and make a table that summarizes the information in the paragraph. Give your table a title.

Fiona read three books over the summer. Trevor read five books over the summer and Chris read two more than Trevor.

33. CREATE DIRECTIONS

Write directions to create the following diagram.

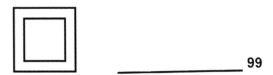

Test your directions by reading them to someone who hasn't seen the drawing. If you need to, improve your directions.

34. WORD WORK

Think of a word that starts with B and write it horizontally in the space below. Now look at the final letter of your word and think of a word that begins with that letter. Write your second word vertically, using the already written letter as the starting point.

35. GRID

Put your pencil on the number 24.

Draw a line to number 16.

Draw a line up two squares.

Now draw a line down 4 squares.

What number is two squares to the right?

4	1			7
16			24	
	8			
		11	17	

36. SECRET LETTER

Use the following statements to identify the secret letter in the table below. As you read each rule, cross out the incorrect letters.

1. I am not in the first row.
2. I am not a vowel.
3. I am not in the word in the word PRINCE.
4. I am not beside P.

What letter am I? _____

ZBAW
KOLP
RUEN

37. COUNTING

Count the number of windows in the room. In the space below, draw one square for each window. Put the letter W in each square.

38. CONDITIONAL

If you like apple pie, draw a picture of yourself eating one. If you don't like apple pie, draw a picture of something you can see right now.

Draw a circle around your drawing and write your name below the circle. Underline your name.

39. CREATE DIRECTIONS

Write directions to create the following diagram.

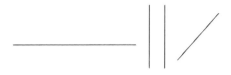

Test your directions by reading them to someone who hasn't seen the drawing. If you need to, improve your directions.

40. DRAWING

Draw a cat. Next put a collar on the cat. Draw the cat's food bowl and favorite toy. Write the cat's name above your drawing. Write your own name below the drawing.

41. ALPHABET

List five shapes on the left hand side of the page. Next, rewrite the list alphabetically in the middle of the page. Next, on the right hand side of the page, rewrite the list in order of the number of sides each shape has.

42. CALENDAR

Draw an apple on the day that is a week after July 1st. Draw a smiley face two days after that. If the apple is on an even date, draw a banana on July 24. If the smiley face is on an odd date, draw a circle on July 20.

JULY

		1	2	3	4	5
6	7	8	9	10	11	12
13	14	15	16	17	18	19
20	21	22	23	24	25	26
27	28	29	30	31		

43. DIRECTIONS

Write your name in the middle of the space below in capital letters. Circle each vowel. Put a square around your name. Draw a triangle under the square. Look around the room and write the name of something you can see that is brown at the bottom of the page.

44. LINES

Use the lines below. On the top line, write the day of the week on the left and your name on the right.

On the third line, write the name of something you can see that is blue.

Circle all the vowels on line three.

Put your initials at the bottom of the page in the middle.

_____

_____

_____

_____

45. OBSERVE

How many doors are in the room where you are now? Add 5 to that number. What number do you end up with? Write it down in the middle of the space below. Put your name at the bottom left and your age at the bottom right.

46. DESCRIPTION

Think about your favorite activity. Write a description about it that is at least 3 sentences long. Make sure to explain why you like that activity.

47. DRAW & DESCRIBE

Find something white in the room where you are. Draw a picture of it. Write three sentences about that object. Number each sentence. Check you have used capitals and punctuation.

48. SHAPES

Draw a vertical line. On the right of the line, write the name of a color. On the left of the line, write the name of an animal. Draw an arrow that goes from the color to the animal.

49. IMAGINE

Your cat has a secret. What is it? Write 3-5 sentences about your cat's secret.

50. PATTERN

Write the next three letters in this pattern. Write the fourth and the sixth letters of the pattern in the space below. On the right, write a word that contains these two letters.

AABBAABBAABBAABB_ _ _

__ __

51. ADD TO

Copy the following sentence, but change the time. Next add another two sentences to continue the story.

Greg arrived at the cinema ten minutes after the movie started.

52. RANDOM WORDS

Make a list of five random words to do with plants.

Now make five different sentences. Each sentence must contain one of the random words and the word BECAUSE.

53. DRAW MAP

Draw a floorpan of your house. If your house has more than one level, choose the level with your bedroom. Label each room and show where the doors are. Include the major furniture or fixtures in each room.

54. CREATE TABLE

Read the following paragraph and make a table that summarizes the information in the paragraph. Give your table a title.

Three people got on the bus at Topham Hill and five people got off. Seven people got off at Fenton Station and two got on. At the last stop, Greenway Mall, three people got off.

55. INFORMATION RETRIEVAL

List four body parts and put two bullet points next to each describing something you know about that body part.

Give your information a title and put your name on the top left.

56. LETTERS

Write 5 letters down the left hand side of the space below. Each letter should be different - no repeats. Think of an animal that starts with each letter and write the animal names in a line at the bottom. Draw a line from each letter to the animal that starts with that letter.

57. MAKE PATTERN

Write the next five numbers in the sequence that matches this rule. The first two number have been written for you.

Start at 34 and decrease by 3.

34, 32, ___, ___, ___, ___, ___

58. WACKY

Write your first and last name in reverse in the space below. For example, the name BEN would be written NEB.

58. MOUSE

Write directions for how the mouse will get to the cheese. Use words like up, down, left, right and tell how many squares to move in each direction. You must avoid the obstacles.

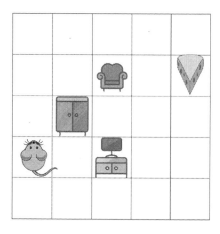

59. DRAW

Write step-by-step instructions for drawing this tree. Try reading your instructions to someone else and see what they draw.

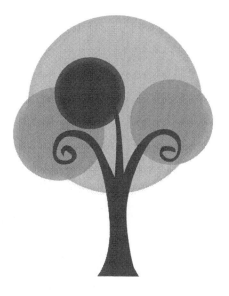

60. CHANGES

Write out the number below, but make the following changes. Subtract 1 from all odd numbers. Subtract 2 from all even numbers.

5 8 3 8 9 1 7 5 3 2 7

– – – – – – – – – – –

Add up all the numbers that you wrote and write the total here.

61. WORD PROBLEM

Write a math word problem about a boy named John who starts with 10 apples and then loses some.

62. CATEGORIZE

Categorize these words into three columns. Put a heading at the top of each column to describe the words in each column.

Animal Beast Alligator Cat Cream Bandage Crowd Anchor Bridge Cast

63. COMPARISON

Look at the table below and write two sentences about sports that have something in common (something the same.)

Now write two sentences about differences between the some of the sports.

Number your sentences.

Sport	Ball?	Team?
Tennis	Yes	No
Ice Hockey	No	Yes
Soccer	Yes	Yes
Skiing	No	No

64. FORMS

Read the paragraph and fill in the form below.

> My Name is Kerry Peterson and I am applying for a job as a waitress in a restaurant. I have previously worked in a coffee shop for two months and I also helped my aunt in her bakery last summer. In both jobs I was responsible for helping customers, taking orders and keeping the shop tidy.

Name: _____

Job You Are Applying For:_____

List your previous work experience:

_____

_____

_____

_____

65. DISTRIBUTION

You have to do 5 math lessons per week, 5 reading lessons per week and 5 science lessons per week. Each lesson takes one hour.

Write out how you will schedule your days from Monday to Friday. Explain your choices.

66. FIND THE PROBLEM

Which instruction is incorrect? Replace it with a correct instruction.

1. Draw a six-point star.
2. Draw a circle around the star.
3. Color in the space outside the star but inside the circle.

67. DRAW

Write step-by-step instructions for drawing this house. Try reading your instructions to someone else and see what they draw.

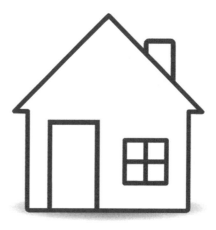

68. MOUSE

Write directions for how the mouse will get to the cheese. Use words like up, down, left, right and tell how many squares to move in each direction. You must avoid the obstacles.

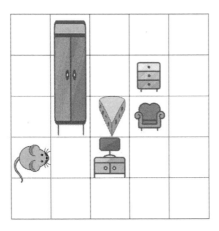

69. CHANGES

Write out the number below, but make the following changes. Divide all even numbers by 2. Add 1 to each odd number except 9.

5 8 3 8 9 1 7 5 3 2 7

- - - - - - - - - - -

Add up all the numbers that you wrote and write the total here.

70. MAKE PATTERN

Write the first seven elements in the sequence that matches this rule.

Start at 2 and increase by the last number plus 1.

71. CONDITIONAL

If your birthday is in summer, draw a picture of you on the beach. If your birthday is spring, draw a picture of you picking flowers. If your birthday is in fall, draw a picture of you raking leaves. If your birthday is in winter, draw a picture of you sliding down the snow.

Write your name in capital letters below your drawing. Give your drawing a title and write it above your picture.

72. CATEGORIZE

Categorize these words into two columns. Put a heading at the top of each column to describe the type of words in each column.

Next, think of a way to categorize these words into two groups according to length. Write the words again under the new headings.

Orange Pumpkin Apple Strawberry Kale Squash Banana Potato Carrot Peach

73. COMPARISON

Write three sentences that compare the clothes listed in the table. Comparisons are when you talk about what is the same and what is different.

Number your sentences. Check for correct spelling, capitalization and punctuation.

Clothes	Season	Body Part
Shorts	Summer	Legs
Long pants	Winter	Legs
Sun hat	Winter	Head
Sandals	Summer	Feet

74. IMAGINE

You get to plan your perfect meal. Describe your meal below. Include what you eat, where you are eating and who you are with.

75. ADD TO

Change the name, age and profession of the person in this sentence. Add three more sentences that talk about why this person wants to change jobs.

John was a 32 year old carpenter, but he wanted to be a rocket scientist.

76. CREATE TABLE

Read the following paragraph and make a table that summarizes the information in the paragraph. Give your table a title.

Liam went to the fruit store and bought six apples and two oranges. Sara bought five apples and three bananas. Peter bought five bananas. Kristy bought ten oranges and four peaches.

Below the table, write how many pieces of fruit were bought altogether.

77. LETTERS

Write 5 letters down the left hand side of the space below. Each letter should be different - no repeats. Think of a sport that starts with each letter. If you can't think of a sport for a particular letter, cross that letter out and write another one next to it. Write the names of the sports on the right hand side of the space below. Draw a wriggly line from each letter to its matching sport.

78. WACKY

Write the word CREATIVE so that it appears correctly when you look at it in a mirror. Use the space below.

79. DISTRIBUTION

You have 3 candy bars, 4 chocolate bars and two ice cream cones.

You like chocolate the best. Jim doesn't like chips. Mia likes everything.

Write down how you will share out the food between the three of you. Explain your choices.

80. WORD PROBLEM

Read the word problem and then write the answer below. If your birthday date is a number smaller than this, draw a circle below the number. If your birthday date is equal to or larger than this number, draw a square below the number.

Katy has ten blocks and Susie gives her five more. How many blocks does Katy have?

81. DRAW MAP

Draw a map of your neighborhood. Include at least 3 streets or roads and label them. Show where your house is. Draw an arrow to show the direction of the nearest shop.

82. OBSERVE

Make a list of the things that you are touching right now. Include everything that any part of your body touches. Put the items in two categories: hard and soft. Make sure to label each category.

83. PATTERN

Create a pattern that uses the letters A B and C. The sixth and seventh members of the pattern must be B C. Write the first nine members of the pattern.

___ ___ ___ ___ ___ _B_ _C_ ___ ___

84. COUNTING

Count the number of chairs in the room. Draw a triangle and write the number of chairs below the triangle. Above the triangle, write the word 'chair'. Draw a circle around everything you have drawn.

85. ALPHABET

Write the first ten letters of the alphabet down the left hand side of the page. Find an adjective that begins with each letter. An adjective is a word that describes something, like *small, pretty, terrific,* etc.

86. SECRET LETTER

Use the following statements to identify the secret number in the table below. As you read each rule, cross out the incorrect numbers.

1. I am neither below 10 nor above 20.
2. I am an even number.
3. I can be divided by 7.

12 - 21 - 31 - 5

6 - 14 - 8 - 15

37 - 28 - 9 - 18

Secret Number____

87. DESCRIPTION

Think about your favorite animal. Write a description of that animal without using the name of the animal. Read the description to an adult or friend and see if they can guess what animal it is.

88. WORD WORK

Think of a word that starts with D and write it horizontally in the space below, starting close to the left.

Now look at the final letter of your word and think of a word that begins with that letter. Write your second word vertically, using the already written letter as the starting point.

Now look at the final letter of your second word and think of a third word that begins with that letter. Write the word horizontally, using the final letter of the second word as the starting point.

Write today's date at the bottom of the page.

89. DRAWING

Design and draw a book cover. Be sure to include the title and author of the book. The cover should include at least one picture.

90. GRID

Start on the number 12.

Draw a line to number 23.

Go left two, down two and right three squares.

Go to the nearest number. What is it?

4	1			7
12			23	
16				
	8			
		11	17	

91. CREATE DIRECTIONS

Write directions to create the following diagram.

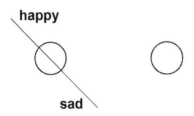

Test your directions by reading them to someone who hasn't seen the drawing. If you need to, improve your directions.

92. CALENDAR

Draw squares on four different days. All the days must be at least 5 days apart.

JULY

		1	2	3	4	5
6	7	8	9	10	11	12
13	14	15	16	17	18	19
20	21	22	23	24	25	26
27	28	29	30	31		

93. DIRECTIONS

Write a 4-word sentence on the bottom half of this page. Count the number of letters in the sentence and write the total above the sentence. If the number is even, draw a large triangle at the top of the space below. If the number is odd, draw a large square at the top of the space below.

94. LINES

Write three words that start with the letter T on the first three lines. On the next three lines, write three words that start with the letter S. Count how many times you have used the letter A and write that on the seventh line.

_____

_____

_____

_____

_____

_____

_____

95. RANDOM WORDS

Think of a word that contains eight or more letters. Write the word at the top of the space below. Next, see if you can come up with five words made from some or all of the letters in the word you thought of. Each word must have three or more letters. Write the words in a column below the original word.

For example, from the word the INFORMATION, you can make NOT, FORM, INTO, etc.

96. DRAW & DESCRIBE

Draw something that doesn't exist. After you have finished drawing, describe what it is and what it is for.

97. INFORMATION RETRIEVAL

Choose a topic and write five interesting things about that topic. Use bullet points. Make sure to add a title and a sentence that explains why the topic is interesting to you.

98. SHAPES

Draw a long horizontal line. On top of the line at the right, write the word 'happy'. Below the line on the right, draw a happy face. Above the line at the left, write the word 'sad'. Below the line on the left, draw a sad face. Put a mark on the line to show how you are feeling now. Write one sentence below the line to explain why you are feeling like that.

99. FIND THE PROBLEM 3

Which instruction is incorrect? Replace it with a correct instruction.

1. Draw a small circle and color it black.
2. Draw another circle around the smaller circle.
3. Draw an oval around the two circles. Make the ends of the oval pointy on the left and right sides.
4. Color inside the second circle.

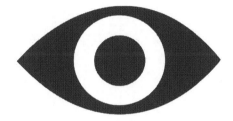

100. ADD TO

Write out the following sentence with these changes.

1. Add a word that describes how the dog barked.
2. Add a word that describes how the dog ran.

Barking, the dog ran after John.

101. SHAPES

Draw three vertical lines spread out across the page. Make sure they are the same length. Between the first two lines, write the letter A upside down. Between the second two lines, write the number 24. Draw a line that connects the top of the first and second vertical lines. Draw a line that connects the bottom of the second and third vertical lines.

102. DIRECTIONS

Draw a square in the middle of the space below and shade it lightly.
Draw a small triangle below it and cover it with stripes. Draw a large
circle about both shapes. Add petals to the circle to make it look like a
flower.

103. CALENDAR

Draw a circle on the calendar three days before July 7th. Draw another one two weeks later than the first circle. Draw a flower three days before the end of the month. If there is more than ten days between a circle and the flower, draw the letter Y on July 22. If not, put the Y on July 23.

JULY

		1	2	3	4	5
6	7	8	9	10	11	12
13	14	15	16	17	18	19
20	21	22	23	24	25	26
27	28	29	30	31		

105. DESCRIPTION

What is the softest thing in the room where you are? Write the name of that thing in the space below. Below the name, write the names of two other soft things. Put the words in alphabetical order and number them.

Choose one of the items and write a description about it. You must include what it looks like and feels like. If appropriate, also describe how it smells, tastes or sounds.

105. DRAW MAP

Draw a rough map of the country of your choice. Locate and label the capital city. Locate and label three other cities or places of interest. You may need to use an atlas or the internet. If so, get the permission of an adult first.

BEFORE YOU GO

If you found this book useful, please leave a short review on your preferred online book store. It makes an amazing difference for independent publishers like Happy Frog Press. Just two sentences will do!

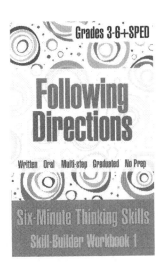

Don't forget to look for other workbooks in the **Six-Minute Thinking Skills** series, publishing in 2018 & 2019.

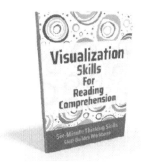

Your learners might also benefit from our **Six-Minute Social Skills series**.

The workbooks in this series build core social skills for kids who have social skills challenges, such as those with Autism, Asperger's and ADHD.

Although numbered, these books can be used in any order.

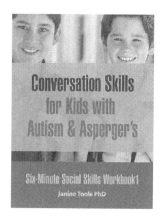

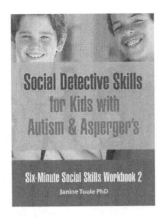

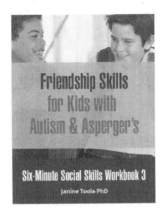

CERTIFICATE

OF

ACHIEVEMENT

THIS CERTIFICATE IS AWARDED TO

_____

IN RECOGNITION OF

_____

_____   _____

DATE   SIGNATURE

101

97